Fit to Surf

The Surfer's Guide to Strength Training & Conditioning

Rocky Snyder, C.S.C.S.

Edited by Dana Brown
Designed by Rocky Snyder
Principal Photography by Rocky Snyder
Additional Photography by Boots McGhee

First published in the U.S.A. in 2001 by Emerson Publishing Company
551 37ᵗʰ Avenue, Santa Cruz, California 95062
Phone: (831) 479-0867
Email: drsnyder@dellnet.com

Library of Congress Card Number: 00-110325
Fit To Surf
The Surfer's Guide To Strength Training & Conditioning
Snyder, Rocky
ISBN 0-9706120-0-1

Printed in the U.S.A.

Table of Contents

Acknowledgements

This book would not have been possible had it not been for my family, friends, and clients who continually urged and supported me to follow through with an idea. Although I can not list everyone involved, my thanks go out to you all.

There are a few people, however, that were directly responsible for helping me see this project through to the end. My wife Dana, who broke me of my procrastinating ways, and Chris Miske, for his ideas and bearing with me through lengthy photo shoots. Kathy Pearlberg, for adding the feminine touch. I would also like to thank Janice and Wingnut Weaver, for introducing me to the world of surfing, and the M10 surf team for letting me use them as guinea pigs during the creation of this book.

FOREWORD

Surfing has undergone a phenomenal period of growth in the past 10 years. New surfers are discovering the lure of the water and the adrenaline rush of dropping in on a wave. Older surfers are returning to the ocean to find the stoke they once had when they were mere groms. Young, old, new surfer or veteran, everyone is having fun in the water.

Surfing is a strenuous sport that requires physical stamina, delicate skill, and balance. Unlike surfing, other sports, such as running and cycling, have measurable indicators to help you determine when you are improving. Being a competitive surfer and rugby player, I recognize the value of fitness for surfing. As surfers, we can no longer ignore the importance of cross training to improve our surfing. Most veteran surfers acknowledge that the most difficult part of learning to surf is actually catching the wave. Historically, many surfers were true watermen, who, not only surfed, but also swam, paddled, bodysurfed and snorkled.

Rocky's book, Fit to Surf, comes at a time when training for surfing is much needed. The new surfer may only get out in the water a couple of times a week, requiring him or her to find other times and places to train. Even if you surf nearly everyday, you should be running, stretching and performing these exercises to make you a better surfer.

Rocky provides a number of illustrated exercises designed to increase strength, skill, and balance. In addition, you will find that these exercises will help prevent injuries and allow you to enjoy surfing even more. We all want to surf more. When you're physically fit to surf, you can catch more waves, stay out longer without getting tired, and perform new and more demanding maneuvers. With a little time, determination and focus you will see improvements in your surfing. Good luck and aloha!

Kevin Miske

CHAPTER 1: INTRODUCTION

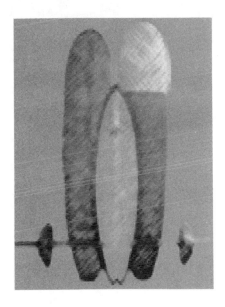

Today people of all ages are surfing and with each year the numbers keep increasing. Improvements in wet suits, equipment and leash cords have allowed people to spend as much time in the waves as they want.

However in today's world, the increase in sedentary lifestyle leads to less active individuals. The combination of reduced activity levels and longer surfing sessions lead to an increase of surf-related injuries of the neck, shoulders, back, hips, and knees.

The young surfers of yesteryear are now grown adults with office jobs and long commutes. Most are not able to surf as much as they used to. Although their minds have remained young, their bodies have aged and have grown accustomed to the reduction of surf sessions. Meanwhile, today's young surfers are sitting behind computers and video games and watching surf videos over and over on their VCR's. The average activity level is less than their mothers and fathers at their age.

These factors lead to the weekend warrior syndrome: People that experience injuries because they are not very active through the week yet they play hard on the weekends. Therefore, there is a need for a conditioning program for surfers to increase strength, endurance and flexibility.

This book is designed to fight the weekend warrior syndrome, to reduce the chance of injury and to strengthen and condition the surfer in a safe and effective manner. Even if most of us are members of health clubs the type of workout programs we perform are not specific to surfing. The programs are not necessarily bad, but they could be better created to improve balance, surfing ability, reduce the chance of injury and combat the physiological effects a sedentary lifestyle can produce.

I have always been involved with athletics ever since I was a kid. Being born and raised in New England, where the seasons change every three months, I found myself competing in many different sports. However, the one thing I never experienced until moving to Santa Cruz, California, was surfing.

The ironic part to this story is that I spent my summers at Hampton Beach, New Hampshire (one of the best beach breaks in New England). To add to this, there was a classic longboard in the basement of my Massachusetts home that was not used since the sixties!

In 1991, I moved to Santa Cruz and immediately fell in love with California. Within a short time, I got hired at a local health club and began my career as a personal fitness trainer.

It is at this time I feel that I must make a confession and an apology. I confess, when I first encountered the surfing community of Santa Cruz, I thought they were just a bunch of people that did nothing all day but stand on the cliffs and watch the waves. It was not until I experienced the love of wave riding that I later learned this was far from the truth.

Prejudices are based on ignorance and I, unfortunately, found I was creating ignorant opinions based on a small stereotypical group. For this, I deeply apologize to the entire surfing community. The surfers I have befriended are the most generous, caring and friendly people I have ever met.

While working at the health club I befriended one member in particular. Her name was Janice, the wife of Robert "Wingnut" Weaver (of Endless Summer II fame). In the fall of that year, for a birthday present, Janice and Wingnut took me surfing at Pleasure Point. At the time I did not think much of the idea except that it might be fun. Little did I know that that day would change my life forever. We paddled out to a small point break and by the time we reached the spot my arms were completely thrashed. Here I thought I was in great shape by working out at least two hours every day. Old overweight guys and little wahines were paddling circles around me. After catching my breath and feeling my burning arms recover, Wingnut turned to me and said, "Here comes your wave. Turn around and paddle. When you feel the wave pick you up, get up on the board." That was the extent of his instructions (or that's all I heard). I started paddling toward the shore as I felt the wave lift me up. He gave me a push down the face, I popped up on my feet and rode the wave straight in until it backed off fifty feet later. Wow! Awesome! What a sensation! My first wave!

Since then, there is hardly a day that passes that I do not stand on the cliff and check out the conditions or listen to the buoy reports. My tide book is always within reach. I quit my job at the health club to open my own athletic center at Pleasure Point, right beside the Santa Cruz Surf Shop. I live a hundred yards from the waves and my quiver has grown to consist of nine boards, from a 6'6" to the 10'0" classic that was in my Massachusetts home. I now train clients in the morning and in the evenings then surf in the afternoons and on the weekends. I find that I have become one of those people that I had made fun of in my ignorant years.

What was curious to me was that all my years of strength training and conditioning did not help much through my first experiences with the winter swells in Santa Cruz. While fighting through overhead sets, after getting caught inside, I felt like I was out of my league. It was only after I looked at how I was training that I realized I was not training to be a stronger surfer but, instead, more like a bodybuilder.

As I mentioned before, when we workout at our local health club the programs that most of us follow focuses more on a bodybuilder's routine than a surfer's. The typical program concentrates on a couple of muscle groups one day and other groups the next. Surfing requires the entire body to work in a synergistic fashion. Therefore, the workout needs to reflect this and be more sport-specific,

A couple of years ago I was invited to vacation on a pleasure craft off the coast of Sumatra. We would spend fifteen days travelling to fifteen of the most fertile surf spots the world had to offer. So several months before we were to leave I set a personal goal of conditioning myself to be in the best surfing shape I could achieve. Using the knowledge I acquired through the National Strength & Conditioning Association, I sat down and analyzed the biomechanics of surfing. What muscles were used the most? What energy system did the muscles utilize? What were the most common injury sites? Once I figured this out I created a conditioning program to help me reach my goal. I trained hard with this program for several months and felt that I was really close to being in the best surf shape of my life.

Unfortunately, Indonesia caught on fire: not just one area but practically every island. Planes were crashing. Boats were colliding and villages were being evacuated. It turned into one of the biggest man-made ecological disasters in history! Needless to say, we did not go, but at least I was ready for the next winter swells in Santa Cruz.

Since then, I have trained many surfers with this program. **It is designed for all surfers, regardless of sex, age or fitness level.** You do not have to be a member of a health club for this program to be effective. Many exercises can be done at home or in the water.

The following chapters will detail exercises and stretches and give the reader sample conditioning programs and information on how to create their own personal surfer's conditioning program. A workout log is provided to record your progress.

There are a few rules that everyone needs to follow:

🏃 The first is that before beginning any new exercise program it is strongly recommended that the participant consult their primary care provider.

🏃 The second rule is to execute proper form during all exercises and stretches. If the form is incorrect it means different muscles are compensating. The more compensation occurs, the higher potential of injury.

🏃 The third rule is if you experience dizziness, pain or discomfort stop immediately.

🏃 The fourth and final rule is to have fun!

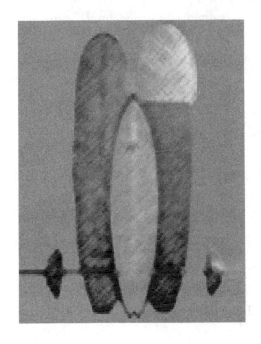

CHAPTER 2:
STRENGTH
TRAINING

Strength training has long been held to be beneficial to increasing an individual's fitness level. Some other benefits of strength training include:

- Increased energy levels.
- Reduced injury potential.
- Increased bone density.
- Increased body circulation.
- Heightened kinesthetic awareness.

When performing strength exercises it is important to remember the five R's. The five R's are elements of every strength program and they are as follows:

1. **Resistance** – The amount of weight or resistance used during an exercise when maintaining proper form.

2. **Repetitions** – The number of times a movement is performed during a set of an exercise. Typically the lower the repetitions (with high resistance) the more basic strength is trained. The higher the repetitions (with low resistance) the more muscular endurance is trained.

3. **Range of Motion** – The movement a muscle is responsible for. Ideally it is best to train the muscle's fullest range of motion.

4. **Rest** – The amount of time spent resting between each set of an exercise. An ideal time frame would be between thirty seconds to two minutes. The more intense the set is, the longer the rest period.

5. **Recovery** – The amount of time spent between strength training workouts of the same muscle group. It has been recommended that 48 hours should be given before strength training the same muscle group. However, this is

not written in stone. If you find that you are strength training the same muscle groups two days in a row it would be wise to change the selection of exercises for the following day (i.e. performing the bench press on Monday and performing push-ups on Tuesday).

Strength Training Exercises

Some of the following exercises require a workout facility with ample space to execute safely but other exercises can be performed at home. **Therefore, as stated before, if you are not a member of a gym you can still create an effective program.**

When strength training remember to try to achieve temporary muscle fatigue in one set of each exercise. Temporary muscle fatigue occurs when the muscles are so exhausted that another repetition can not be performed with proper form. **It is important that proper form occur from start to finish in a set.** It is equally important to have someone act as a spotter when performing exercises with weights that are suspended over or above the body. **If you experience pain when performing an exercise stop immediately and omit that exercise from your workout for the time being.**

Push Up on the Knees

This is a good way for the beginner to perform the exercise.

- ⚘ Hands should be placed in a parallel position just outside shoulder width.

- ⚘ Support the body on the hands and knees.

- ⚘ Breathe in on the descent and breathe out when pushing up.

- ⚘ Lower the body until the chest barely touches the floor or until the elbows form a ninety-degree angle.

- ⚘ Keep the body rigid by contracting the abdominal muscles.

- ⚘ Do not allow the back to arch or bow at any time.

Major muscles involved: Pectorals, Deltoids, and Triceps.
Relevance: Strengthens upper body for pop ups.

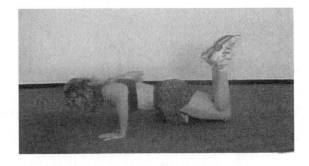

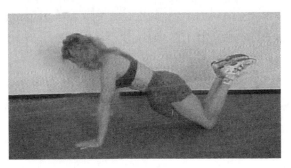

Push Up on the Toes

This position is more demanding than push-ups on the knees.

⚡ Hands should be placed in a parallel position just outside shoulder width.

⚡ Support the body on the hands and toes.

⚡ Breathe in on the descent and breathe out when pushing up.

⚡ Lower the body until the chest barely touches the floor or until the elbows form a ninety-degree angle.

⚡ Keep the body rigid by contracting the abdominal muscles.

⚡ Do not allow the back to arch or bow at any time.

Major muscles involved: Pectorals, Deltoids, and Triceps.
Relevance: Strengthens upper body for pop ups.

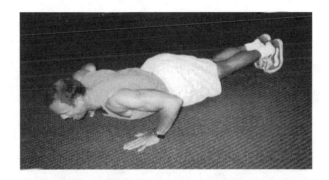

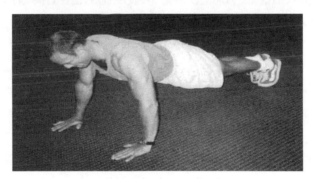

Push Up on the Balance Board

For this type of push-up a device called a balance board is needed. It can be purchased or easily made.

- The balance board is a square piece of plywood twenty inches by twenty inches with two semi-circular pieces of wood screwed into the bottom of the board.

- This allows the board to wobble from side to side. This wobbling effect is similar to popping up on a surfboard and helps to train the body to be more balanced when exerting force.

- When performing push-ups on the balance board it may be a good idea to start on the knees before performing the exercise on the toes.

- Perform a push up with the same form as described in the previous pages.

Major muscles involved: Pectorals, Deltoids, and Triceps.
Relevance: Enhances coordination for pop-ups.

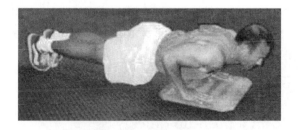

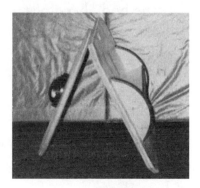

Two Types Of Balance Boards

Plyometric Push Up
on Balance Board

This is one of the more advanced ways to perform the push-up. This exercise will train the muscles to respond quickly and powerfully to propel the body off the floor.

⚞ Begin with hands on the balance board.

⚞ Perform a push-up quickly.

⚞ So quick that the body becomes weightless.

⚞ Allow the hands to lift off the board and quickly land on the floor on either side of the balance board.

⚞ Quickly perform another push-up so the body is again weightless and return the hands back on to the balance board.

(It may be a good idea to first perform this exercise on the knees before advancing to the toe position.)

Major muscles involved: Pectorals, Deltoids, and Triceps.
Relevance: Trains upper body to be quick & explosive.

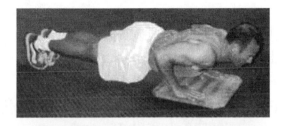

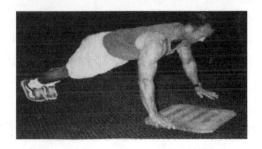

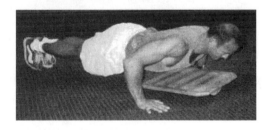

Bench Press

🏊 Lie on a flat bench.

🏊 Hold a dumbbell in each hand or grip a barbell with hands placed at just outside shoulder width.

🏊 Support the dumbbells, or bar, with straight arms, above the shoulders.

🏊 Inhale as the dumbbells, or bar, lowers to a point above the middle of the chest (elbows should be at right angles).

🏊 Exhale as the weight is pressed upward to the starting position.

Major Muscles Involved: Pectorals, Deltoids, Triceps.
Relevance: Strengthens Pop-up muscles.

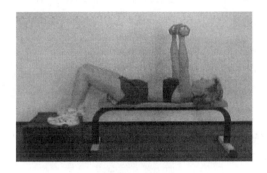

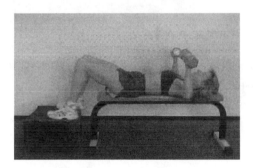

Bench Dip

🏊 Place both hands, shoulder width apart, on the front edge of a bench, chair or box.

🏊 Straighten the arms so the body weight is supported.

🏊 Inhale as the elbows bend and the body lowers so the elbows and shoulders are the same height.

🏊 Exhale as the body is pushed upward to the starting position.

🏊 Start this exercise with the feet on the floor.

🏊 To increase the intensity place both heels up on another chair, bench, or box.

Major muscles involved: Pectorals, Deltoids, and Triceps.
Relevance: Strengthens paddling muscles.

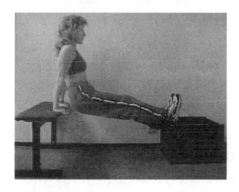

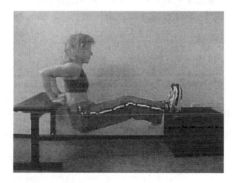

Lat Pulldown

⚡ The body can be positioned on one knee and one foot rather than sitting. The knee and foot position helps promote balance while strengthening the upper body.

⚡ Exhale as the bar is pulled below the chin and inhale on the return.

⚡ Keep the torso as still as possible while pulling up and down. Any extra body movement will incorporate other muscles than the ones that are being targeted.

⚡ The bar may be gripped in a number of ways: wide grip, narrow grip, and reverse grip. Each grip incorporates a large group of upper body muscles though the concentration may be focused on one muscle more than another depending on the grip. One way is not necessarily better than the other, however, it may be better to alternate between grips from one workout to the next.

Major muscles involved: Latissimus Dorsi, Middle Trapezius, Posterior Deltoid, and Biceps.
Relevance: Strengthens major paddling muscles.

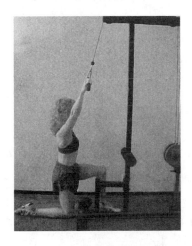

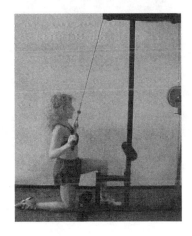

Pull Up

⚴ Grasp a pull up bar with hands shoulder width apart.

⚴ Starting from a straight arm hanging position, exhale as the body is pulled up so the chin is raised above the bar.

⚴ Inhale as the body lowers back to the starting position.

⚴ Be sure not to kick with the legs to try to help raise the body.

Major muscles involved: Latissimus Dorsi, Middle Trapezius, Posterior Deltoid, and Biceps.
Relevance: Strengthens major paddling muscles.

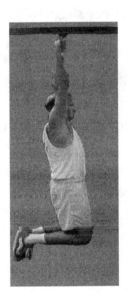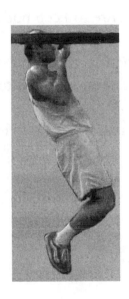

Horizontal Pull Up

⚑ Grasp a bar with both hands shoulder width apart and with feet on the floor in front of the body.

⚑ Be sure to keep both knees slightly bent.

⚑ Keeping the body stiff and straight, exhale as the chest is pulled to the bar.

⚑ Inhale as the body is lowered back to the starting position.

⚑ Be sure to keep the abdominal muscles tight to prevent the back from arching or the hips from sagging.

Major muscles involved: Middle Trapezius, Rhomboids, Posterior Deltoid, and Biceps.

Relevance: Strengthens mid-back paddling muscles.

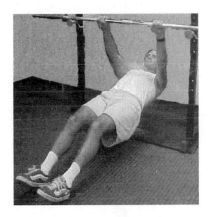

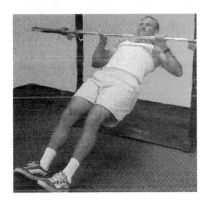

Straight Arm Pulldown

🏄 Stand upright with feet parallel and knees slightly bent.

🏄 Grab the bar with hands shoulder width apart, elbows straight and arms stiff.

🏄 Exhale as the bar is pulled downward to the front of the thighs.

🏄 Inhale as the bar is returned to shoulder height (the arms should be parallel to the floor).

Major Muscles Involved: Pectorals, Latissimus Dorsi, and Triceps.
Relevance: Mimics double arm paddle.

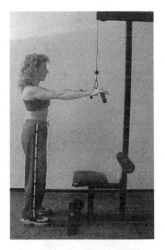

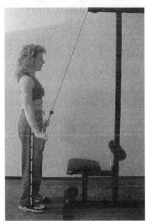

Dumbbell Pullover

✦ Lie face up, parallel or perpendicular on a flat bench.

✦ Grasp a dumbbell with both hands.

✦ Keeping arms slightly bent but stiff, inhale as the arms lower the dumbbell over the head toward the floor.

✦ Once the dumbbell has reached head height, reverse direction and exhale.

✦ Be sure to keep the abdominal muscles contracted to protect the lower back.

✦ Keep both feet firmly planted on the floor or bench.

Major muscles involved: Pectorals, Latissimus Dorsi, Posterior Deltoid, and Triceps.
Relevance: Strengthens paddling muscles.

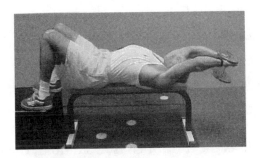

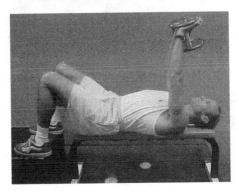

One Arm Row

- 🏄 Place one knee and the hand of the same side on a bench.

- 🏄 The other leg is standing on the floor with the knee slightly bent while the free hand grasps a dumbbell.

- 🏄 The back should be straight and the head in a neutral position.

- 🏄 Exhale as the dumbbell is lifted up to the ribcage.

- 🏄 Inhale as the dumbbell lowers back to a straight arm position.

- 🏄 Repeat exercise using opposite hand and standing on opposite leg.

Major muscles involved: Latissimus Dorsi, Middle Trapezius, Rhomboids, Posterior Deltoid, and Biceps. **Relevance:** Strengthens mid-back for paddling.

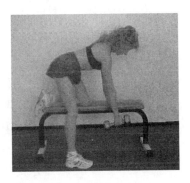

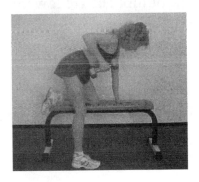

Reverse Dumbbell Fly

⚐ Place feet parallel and placed hip width apart.

⚐ Bend at the waist so the shoulders are slightly above hip height and keep the back straight.

⚐ Grasp a dumbbell in each hand.

⚐ Exhale as the dumbbells are raised upward and out away from the body until the dumbbells are shoulder height.

⚐ Inhale as the dumbbells are lowered back to the starting position.

⚐ Keep the torso as still as possible.

⚐ Do not allow the lower back to lift the torso as the dumbbells are raising.

Major muscles involved: Middle Trapezius, Rhomboids, and Posterior Deltoid.
Relevance: Helps promote shoulder stabilization.

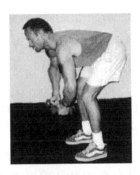

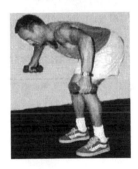

Triceps Pushdown

⚼ Stand upright with feet hip width apart and knees slightly bent.

⚼ Grasp the handle with both hands and pull down so the elbows are nestled beside the rib cage. This is the starting position.

⚼ Exhale as the bar is pushed down to a straight arm position.

⚼ Inhale as the elbows bend and the handle is returned to the starting position.

⚼ Keep the elbows beside the rib cage at all times so the movement only rotates through the elbows.

Major muscles involved: Triceps.
Relevance: Build strong paddling arms.

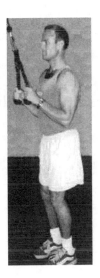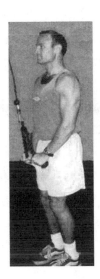

External Rotation

🏄 Lie on one side with the bottom arm folded under the head for support and the legs bent and parallel.

🏄 The upper arm is bent at a right angle with the elbow pressed into the rib cage.

🏄 Hold a dumbbell in that hand and exhale as the dumbbell lifts above the elbow.

🏄 Inhale as the dumbbell is lowered back to the starting position.

Major muscles involved: Rotator cuff muscles.
Relevance: Helps promote shoulder stabilization.

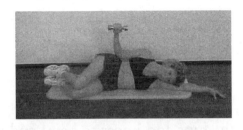

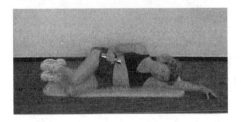

Squat

✦ Stand with feet hip width apart or slightly wider.

✦ Hold dumbbells by the hips or rest a barbell on the shoulders, just above the shoulder blades (not on the neck).

✦ Inhale as the body descends.

✦ Allow the hips and knees to bend and keep the chest upright.

✦ Reverse direction and exhale until the legs are almost straight.

✦ Make sure the hips and shoulders lower and raise at the same time.

✦ Do not allow the hips to descend below the knees.

**Major muscles involved: Gluteals, Hamstrings, and
Quadriceps.
Relevance: Enhances leg strength and balance.**

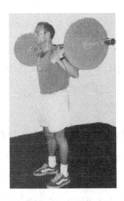

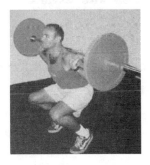

Split Squat

🏄 Stand in a forward split position with the feet two to three feet apart and pointing straight ahead.

🏄 Hold dumbbells by the hips or rest a barbell on the shoulders, just above the shoulder blades (not on the neck).

🏄 Inhale as the body descends until the rear knee is an inch from the floor.

🏄 Reverse direction and exhale until the legs are almost straight.

🏄 Make sure the hips and shoulders lower and raise at the same time.

Major muscles involved: Gluteals, Hamstrings, and Quadriceps.
Relevance: Builds leg strength and balance.

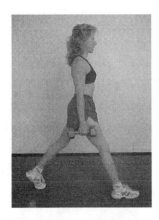

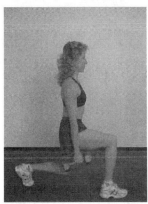

Forward Lunge

The difference between a lunge and a squat is that a squat has a straight up and down movement whereas a lunge has a forward, backward, or lateral movement combined with the up and down movement.

🏃 Stand upright with dumbbells by the hips or rest a barbell on the shoulders, on the top of the shoulder blades (not on the neck).

🏃 Inhale as one foot takes a step forward and the body descends so the hips are parallel with the forward knee.

🏃 Exhale as the forward leg pushes off the floor to return the body back to the starting position.

🏃 Keep the upper body upright at all times.

🏃 Do not allow the shoulders to push back first.

🏃 The movement should originate in the hips and not the lower back.

Major muscles involved: Gluteals, Hamstrings, and Quadriceps.
Relevance: Builds leg strength and balance with change of direction.

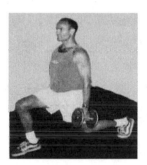
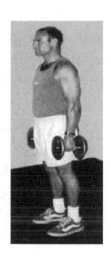

Reverse Lunge

♣ Stand upright with dumbbells by the hips or rest a barbell on the shoulders, on top of the shoulder blades (not on the neck).

♣ Inhale as one foot takes a step backwards and the body descends so the hips are parallel with the forward knee.

♣ Exhale as the rear leg pushes off the floor to return the body back to the starting position.

♣ It is important that the upper body remains upright on the descent and on the return.

♣ <u>Do not</u> allow the shoulders to push forward first.

♣ The movement should originate in the hips and not the lower back.

Major muscles involved: Gluteals, Hamstrings, and Quadriceps.
Relevance: Builds leg strength and balance with change of direction.

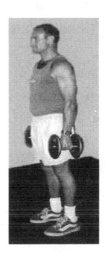
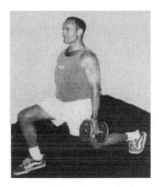

Walking Lunge

🏄 Stand upright with dumbbells by the hips or rest a barbell on the shoulders, above the shoulder blades (not on the neck).

🏄 Inhale as one foot takes a step forward and the body descends so the hips are parallel with the forward knee.

🏄 Exhale as the rear leg pushes off the floor to bring the body forward to a standing position.

🏄 Repeat the movement using the opposite leg to step forward.

🏄 It is important that the upper body remains upright at all times.

🏄 <u>Do not</u> allow the shoulders to push forward first.

🏄 The movement should originate in the hips and not the lower back.

Major muscles involved: Gluteals, Hamstrings, and Quadriceps.

Relevance: Builds leg strength, balance, and coordination.

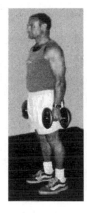 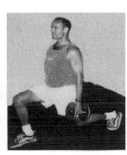 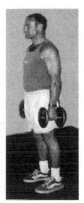

Wall Sit

⚹ Sit against a wall so the lower back is flat and the knees and hips are the same height from the floor.

⚹ Feet are parallel, four inches apart and pointing straight ahead.

⚹ The feet should be away from the wall so the heels are directly below the knees.

⚹ The ankles, knees, and hips should all be at right angles.

⚹ The weight of the body should be pressed through the heels and not the toes.

Major muscles involved: Rectus Femoris.
Relevance: Enhances leg strength and reduces low back tension.

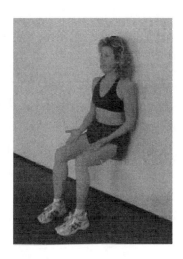

Abdominal Crunch

- Lie face up on the floor with knees bent at right angles and feet flat.
- Clasp hands together and cradle the back of the head.
- Keep the shoulder blades contracted so the elbows stay parallel with the shoulders.
- Exhale as the head, elbows, and shoulders lift off the floor as one object.
- As this occurs the lower back presses into the floor and the abdominal muscles contract.
- Inhale as the body returns to the floor.
- For added intensity, perform the same exercise with the legs raised off the floor above the hips.

Major muscles involved: Rectus Abdominals.
Relevance: Strengthens trunk and stretches low back.

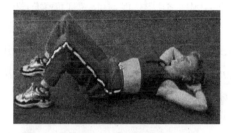

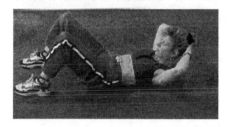

Oblique Crunch

✈ Lie on the floor face up with one knee bent at a right angle and foot flat.

✈ The opposite ankle is crossed over the bent knee.

✈ Cradle one hand under the back of the head and place the opposite arm, palm down, away from the body.

✈ Exhale as the cradled arm lifts off the floor, simultaneously with the same shoulder and the head, in the direction of the crossed leg.

✈ Inhale as the body lowers back to the floor.

✈ Keep the hips and legs as still as possible.

Major muscles involved: Abdominals and Obliques.
Relevance: Strengthens trunk rotation and stretches low back.

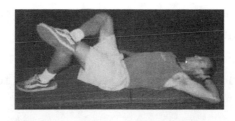

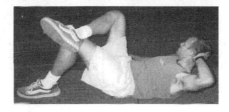

Lower Back Exercise

🏄 Lie face-down with arms outstretched and legs straight.

🏄 Exhale as one leg and the opposite arm lifts off the floor.

🏄 Inhale as the arm and leg lower back to the floor.

🏄 Repeat the movement using opposite limbs.

🏄 Be sure to keep the head facing the floor through the entire exercise.

Major muscles involved: Gluteals, Lower Trapezius and Erector Spinae.
Relevance: Conditions body to strengthen in a prone position.

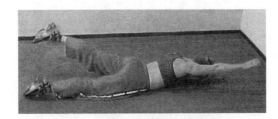

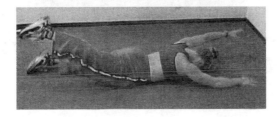

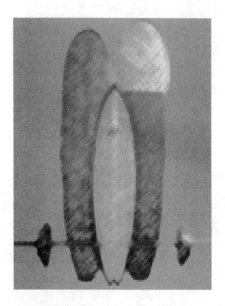

Skill Transfer Exercises

Skill transfer exercises are movements that closely mimic a specific maneuver in a sport or activity. These types of exercises can help if you are looking to: acquire a stronger drop-knee turn, a faster cutback, a deeper bottom turn, a quicker pop up off the board, etc.

The following exercises are suggested for better performance in regards to a specific skill. Select the exercises that will help condition you for the maneuver you want to focus on, and add them to your program.

Reverse Lunge
for
Drop Knee Turn

⚡ Stand upright with dumbbells by the hips or rest a barbell on the shoulders, on top of the shoulder blades (not on the neck).

⚡ Inhale as one foot takes a step backwards and the body descends so the hips are parallel with the forward knee.

⚡ Exhale as the rear leg pushes off the floor to return the body back to the starting position.

⚡ It is important that the upper body remains upright on the descent and on the return.

⚡ Do not allow the shoulders to push forward first. The movement should originate in the hips and not the lower back.

Major muscles involved: Gluteals, Hamstrings, and Quadriceps.

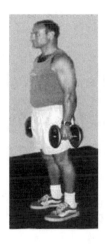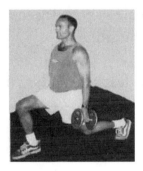

Hanging Leg Lift
for
Off-the-Top

⚐ With upper arms placed in straps hang from a chin up bar, or grasping the bar as if about to perform a pull up.

⚐ Exhale as both legs bend and the feet lift up and to the side.

⚐ The feet should be raised to the same height of the hips.

⚐ Inhale as the legs lower to the starting position.

⚐ Be sure to alternate raises from left to right.

Major muscles involved: Psoas Major, Hip Abductors, and Rectus Abdominals.

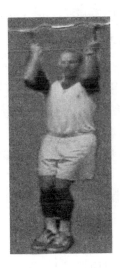
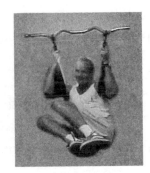

Supine Eagles
for
Bottom Turns

🏄 Lie on the back, with legs straight and arms away from the body with palms down.

🏄 Exhale and lift the left leg up and across the body until the toes touch the right hand.

🏄 Inhale as the leg returns to the starting position.

🏄 Switch legs, bringing the right toes up to the left hand.

🏄 Be sure to keep both shoulders in contact with the floor at all times.

Major muscles involved: Psoas Major, Quadriceps, and Obliques.

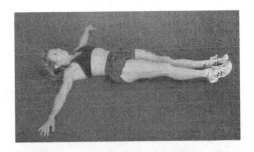

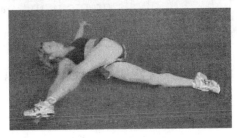

Standing Torso Rotation
for
Stronger Cut Backs

⚞ Stand in a forward split position with legs two to three feet apart.

⚞ Lower the body until the hips are the same height as the front knee.

⚞ Hold light dumbbells or medicine balls (with handles) in each hand.

⚞ Raise the arms away from the body just below shoulder height.

⚞ Rotate through the hips as the arms swing clockwise and then counterclockwise back to the starting position.

⚞ The entire body should rotate at the same time.

Major muscles involved: Low Back, Rectus Abdominals, and Obliques.

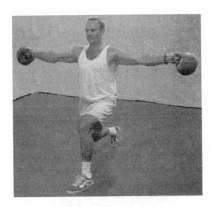

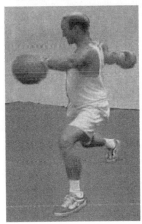

Burpees
For
Quicker Pop Ups

✺ Begin in the downward phase of a push up.

✺ Hands should be placed directly below the shoulders with the body lifted just off the floor.

✺ In one quick move, push off the floor.

✺ Bring both feet forward into a regular or goofy foot stance.

✺ Quickly return back to the starting position and repeat.

Major muscles involved: Pectorals, Deltoids, Triceps, and Psoas Major.

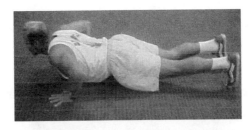

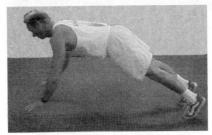

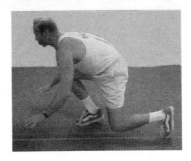

Popping Push Up
for
Stronger Pop Up

✹ Perform a push up on the toes with enough explosive power that the hands lift off the floor.

✹ Lower the body, in a controlled manner, to the downward phase of the push up.

✹ Be sure not to allow the body to lose its rigidity.

✹ <u>Do not</u> let the hips or back sag at any time.

Major muscles involved: Pectorals, Deltoids, and Triceps.

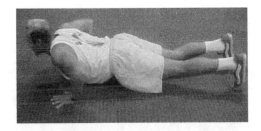

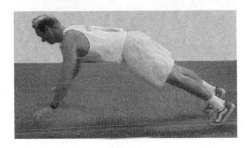

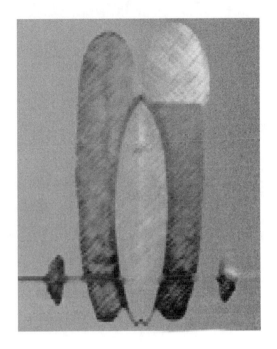

CHAPTER 3:
ENDURANCE
TRAINING

A surfer requires not only strength for strong paddling skills but also the muscular endurance to maintain stamina for an entire surf session. Strength training conditions the body to be strong but it is essential to include endurance training in a surfer's workout to focus on stamina. When creating an effective endurance program there are four elements that must be addressed. Just by increasing one of these elements will increase the demand placed on the body. They are as follows:

🏊 **Frequency** – The number of times the exercise is performed in a length of time.

🏊 **Duration** – The length of time it takes to perform the exercise.

🏊 **Intensity** – The desired effort level performed during the exercise.

🏊 **Type** – The choice of exercise performed in a workout.

The following are cardiovascular exercises that are either sport-specific to surfing or can be performed as cross-training exercises.

Paddling

It may sound obvious, but to become a stronger paddling machine a surfer needs to paddle! A basketball player shoots baskets. A marathon runner runs. There is an element known as the overload principle. The overload principle refers to the method of exhausting muscles to such an extent that physiological adaptations occur with the involved muscles, making them stronger and/or more endurable. An example of this principle would be if a person performed as many push-ups as possible. Sooner or later that individual would grow stronger because their muscles were taxed to a point of muscular fatigue.

The longer a surfboard is the less effort or work is required to paddle. The shorter the surfboard the less buoyancy and the more drag is created so more effort is demanded.

When creating your own paddling program in Chapter 5, you can start out with a longer board and progress to shorter surfboards to increase the workout intensity. Don't worry if you have only one board. There are other ways of increasing your workout intensity.

Resistance Paddling

Purchase a small plastic bucket with a sturdy handle or use a large coffee can. Drill holes in the bucket/can until it looks like Swiss cheese. The more holes you drill the less resistance you will have. The bucket/can can be dragged behind you for added resistance when paddling. Simply connect the handle to the ankle leash.

Partner Paddling

If you have a paddling partner take turns towing each other by holding on to the person's leash. To determine when to change places you can do it in a number of ways:

- Count the number of strokes and switch when you get to a pre-determined amount.
- Wear a watch and establish an interval time of one to five minutes.
- Choose a distance to cover of fifty to a hundred and fifty yards before switching places.

Land Paddle
With Resistance Bands

When the weather is bad and turning the water into nothing but chop but you still want to do a paddle workout, go to a sporting goods store and purchase a rubber resistance band (preferably one with handles). Secure the middle of the band to an immovable object a few feet off the ground. Hold on to both ends of the resistance band and kneel or lay face down on a flat padded bench and mimic the motions of paddling. The further away the bench is placed the more resistance is applied. Be sure to check for wear and tear in the band. Replace it if any tear or abrasion occurs.

Swimming

Swimming is a great cross-training exercise for surfers and if your leash snaps or you're not wearing one, swimming may become very important! It may be a good idea to take a few lessons at your local swim center if you are unfamiliar with proper form.

Underwater Swimming

Surfers need to be able to hold their breath underwater for prolonged periods of time, especially when surfing bigger waves. It is important to train the lungs and the mind to be able to stay underwater, without panicking, while swimming back to the surface. Wear a watch to help keep track of time when performing underwater swims. Start with intervals of fifteen to thirty seconds and slowly add more time with each workout. Be sure to do this close to shore or in a pool for safety reasons.

Stair Climbing

Cross training with health club stair climbing machines can be a good workout. But if there is a long flight of stairs in the neighborhood, hopefully wooden stairs, then try going up and down those for an endurance workout. When climbing make sure the form is the same as when running or walking...stay tall. Be sure to walk slowly on the way down to allow your body and heart rate to recover.

Walking & Running

Whether you walk or run it does not matter, you will reach the same destination eventually. It just might take more time if you walk. They are both healthy choices. Whichever you choose, be sure to be as tall as possible. Keep the head over the shoulders, chest up and hips tucked under. Be sure the arms swing freely forward and that the feet are pointing forward.

Rowing Machine

The rowing machine is a great full body workout and a terrific cross-training exercise. Be sure to have good seated posture at all times. Use the legs as much as possible; they are your biggest muscles. Exhale when pulling the handle inward.

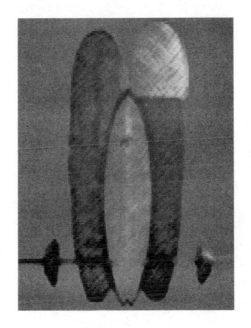

CHAPTER 4:
FLEXIBILITY
TRAINING

One of the most important elements in fitness yet often the most overlooked is flexibility. When muscles are tighter than they should be the body's movement is restricted. This makes any action require more effort. The more often an individual stretches the more flexible that person becomes. Just by taking a few minutes to stretch during your workout or before you surf, the better the body will function.

The longer a stretch is held the more likely the muscles will relax and lengthen. Holding a stretch for ten seconds is good but one minute is better. If any stretch causes pain, stop immediately and omit that stretch from the program for the time being. Not all stretches are for everybody. Perform those stretches that your instinct tells you feels good. **The following stretches can be performed daily.**

Crossed Knee Lift

🏊 Lie on the floor face up with arms out in a cross-like position and palms down.

🏊 Cross one ankle over the opposite knee.

🏊 Lift that knee up directly above the hip and hold for at least fifteen seconds.

🏊 Repeat the stretch using the opposite leg.

Relevance: Stretches hip muscles that tighten, and strengthens other hip muscles that weaken when surfing.

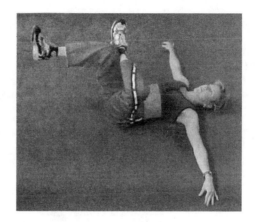

Crossover Twist

⚑ Lie on the floor face up with arms in a cross position and palms down.

⚑ Bend the knees at right angles so the feet are flat.

⚑ Cross one ankle over the opposite knee.

⚑ Keeping the shoulders and arms on the floor, rotate the leg and the crossed foot over to the side until both rest on the floor.

⚑ The leg that is not on the ground should point upward to the sky.

⚑ Hold for at least fifteen seconds.

⚑ Repeat the stretch using the opposite leg and foot.

Relevance: Stretches tight hip and low back muscles, and enhances trunk rotation.

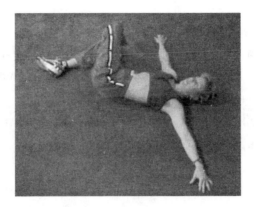

Mad Cat Stretch

🏊 Support the body on all fours with hands directly below the shoulders and knees below the hips.

🏊 Breathe out as the back arches upward and breathe in as the back bows back down.

🏊 The head moves in the opposite direction of the back.

🏊 The movement should be continuous without pausing at the top or bottom.

Relevance: Promotes better movement in the back, shoulders, and hips.

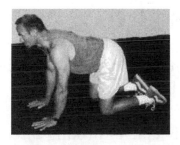

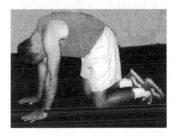

Chest & Shoulder Stretch

↗ Stand with feet parallel and knees slightly bent.

↗ Clasp both hands together with fingers inter-locked behind the back.

↗ Straighten both arms and pull the hands away from the body.

↗ Keep body upright making sure the torso does not bend forward.

Relevance: Stretches muscles that tighten when paddling.

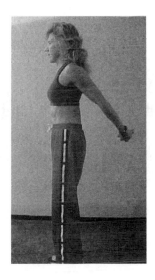

Crossed Arm Stretch

⚞ With elbows bent, cross one arm above the other so that the elbow is nestled in the pit of the opposite arm.

⚞ The hand of the lower arm should grasp the opposite wrist with both arms pointing upward.

⚞ Pull both elbows downward and hold.

⚞ Be sure to switch arms and perform the same stretch.

Relevance: Stretches neck and shoulder muscles that tighten when supporting the head during paddling.

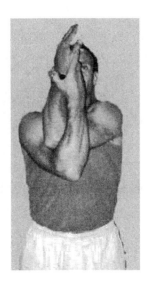

Arm Circles

🏊 Extend arms out by the side of the body at shoulder height.

🏊 Keep the shoulder blades pinched together as the arms make six-inch circles backward with palm face up.

🏊 Flip the palms down and reverse the circle direction.

🏊 Keep the body as still as possible with the movement only occurring at the shoulder joint.

Relevance: Promotes proper shoulder movement for paddling.

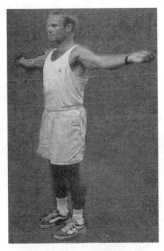

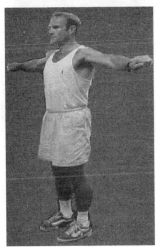

Shoulder Pivots

🏄 Curl the fingers in toward the palms and place the knuckles against the temples with palms faced forward.

🏄 Keeping knuckle contact with the temples <u>at all times.</u>

🏄 Pull the elbows together until they touch and then pull the elbows apart as far as possible.

Relevance: Promotes proper shoulder function when paddling.

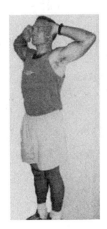 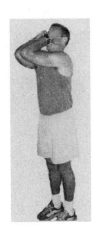

Lateral Neck Stretch

🏄 Place the left arm behind the back with the elbow bent.

🏄 With the right hand, gently pull the left side of the head toward the right shoulder.

🏄 Repeat using opposite arms.

Relevance: Stretches neck muscles that tighten when paddling.

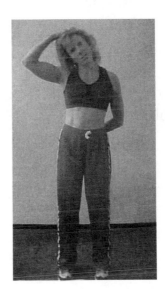

Forward Neck Stretch

🏄 Stand with feet parallel and knees slightly bent.

🏄 With both hands, reach over the head and gently pull the back of the head forward and bend into the neck.

🏄 The chin should lower toward the middle of the clavicles (collarbones).

Relevance: Stretches neck muscles that tighten when paddling.

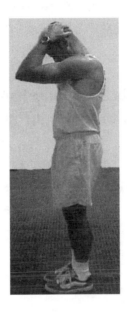

Downward Facing Dog

✴ Start on the hands and knees.

✴ Hands should be below the shoulders and knees below the hips with the toes curled up on the floor.

✴ Push the body back onto the hands and feet with legs, arms, and back straight.

✴ Press the heels to the floor while maintaining straight legs and push the hips away from the hands.

Relevance: Stretches low back, hamstrings, and calf muscles that tighten when surfing.

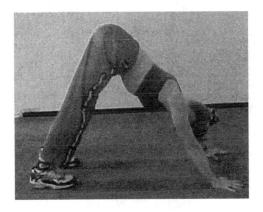

Quadriceps Stretch

🏄 Stand on the left leg and place the left hand of against a wall.

🏄 Bend the right leg at the knee and grasp the roof of the foot with the right hand.

🏄 Be sure to keep both knees parallel and tuck the buttocks downward.

🏄 Repeat with the opposite leg.

Relevance: Reduces hip tension for better balance.

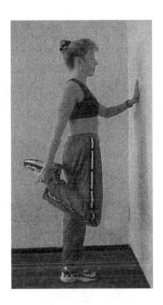

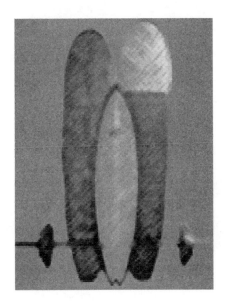

CHAPTER 5:
SURF TEAM
DRILLS

This chapter is devoted to those that coach surf teams. Most of the book focuses on what an individual can do to be a stronger, fitter surfer. But what do you do when you are training a number of surfers at one time? As a coach it is important to build camaraderie which is all the more reason to train as a team. **When strength training, try to pair up team members that have similar strength levels so each can act as a spotting partner.**

The following pages give examples of team conditioning drills that can be performed in the water and on the land. These drills can be scheduled on strength training days or on the off days. They are meant to be challenging yet fun. The only pieces of equipment you may require are surfboards and five cones or flags.

Drafting Paddle

For this drill, choose a distance such as one mile, half mile, or a quarter mile. When beginning this program it may be good to start with a light distance and as they become more conditioned increase the distance. Have the team paddle with one surfer behind the other in a straight line. The lead surfer begins to paddle almost as hard as he/she can with the rest close behind. The last surfer in line has to break away from the line and overtake the leader. As soon as the last surfer takes the lead position the next surfer in the back must battle hard to take the lead. The drill resembles how geese fly south for the winter. The exercise should continue until the desired distance is covered.

Drafting Runs and Cycling

When running or cycling as a team the same drafting technique described above can be used. Have the team form a straight line. The last person must overtake the leader. This should continue until the desired time or distance is reached. For safety purposes choose a route with little or no traffic. It may be a good idea to run on a track or cycle in a park or forest.

Paddle Relays

Break the team up into four groups (A, B, C, and D). Have groups A and B at the starting line and groups C and D positioned fifty to a hundred yards away. Blow a whistle to start the relay. One surfer from group A and another from group B paddle as hard as they can to reach and tag a surfer from group C and D. Once tagged, surfers from C and D paddle as hard as they can to tag surfers in groups A and B. This relay should continue until the last surfer finishes. For added incentive, have the winning team choose a fitting punishment for the losing team (i.e. winners get choice of waves during practice).

Suicide Drills

Set up five cones on the beach in a straight line, ten yards apart, so the total distance is forty yards. Team members have to sprint from the first cone to the second and back to the first. Then sprint to the third cone and back to the first without stopping. Then to the fourth cone and back to the first. Then finally to the fifth cone and finish back at the first. Allow two minutes recovery time before beginning the next set. Perform three to four sets. The same drill can be performed paddling on the water.

Water Sprints

In knee high water have team members sprint twenty to forty yards. Allow one to two minutes recovery time before beginning the next set. Make certain that the running surface is level and free of rocks and reef for safety reasons. This drill can also be done on soft sand or set up as a relay to keep things interesting.

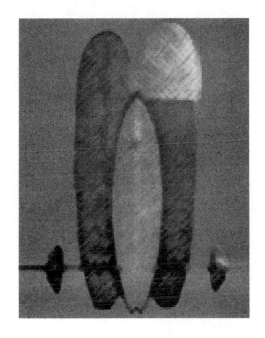

CHAPTER 6:
NUTRITIONAL
GUIDELINES

I am a Certified Strength and Conditioning Specialist, not a registered dietician or certified nutritionist. It would be wise to consult one of those professionals if you are interested in a complete eating plan. Both dieticians and nutritionists can help create an individualized nutritional program.

The following are, more or less, suggestions to living a healthy lifestyle with the foods we eat. Remember the old saying, "You are what you eat", well it is true. Our bodies react to everything we eat and drink. Our bodies are at their best when we feed it what it needs. Our bodies become taxed when we feed it the wrong things.

Most everyone in this country has been raised with foods that the human body has never been introduced to before: candy bars, fast food, ice cream, TV. dinners, most supermarket foods and alcohol (okay, alcohol has been around a long time, but the average consumption level is higher). Let's consider these "new" foods as the foods that are not necessarily the best choice to have as the core of your diet. It might be wiser to build the core of your diet on things like seasonal organic fruits and vegetables, lean cuts of meat and fish, and most seeds and nuts. Most of the foods you want to eat should be that which could have been hunted, caught, gathered from the ground or plucked from a tree.

Here are a few other suggestions you may want to incorporate into diet if you are looking to trim down.

🏊 Eat protein at every meal.

🏊 Cut out wheat and flour based products.

🏊 Don't eat starchy foods for dinner.

🏊 Eat fruit that is low in sugar and high in fiber.

🏊 Limit yourself to two pieces of fruit a day.

🏊 Reduce the amount of dairy products: milk, cheese, and ice cream, etc.

🏊 Drink water! We, as humans, are made up of mostly water, so stay hydrated.

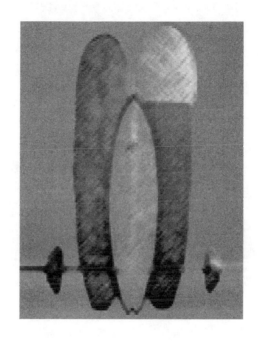

CHAPTER 7: CREATING YOUR PROGRAM

When setting out to create your own conditioning program there are a few things to keep in mind. First, start out slowly and progress on to more intense workouts as your body gets accustomed to these exercises.

Often we find a person who, in the past, has exercised regularly for a long period of time but who has not been exercising in the last few months or years. They often start their new exercise program where they had left off. This can be dangerous because their muscles have de-conditioned even though their egos have remained intact. The chance of injury or extreme muscle soreness is greatly increased in this case. It is important to start out slowly so the body can adapt to the new strain that exercise places on the body.

Secondly, if any sharp pain is experienced while performing an exercise, stop immediately. The exercise may not be the right one for you or the form may be incorrect. In this case, refer back to the description of the exercise to see if it was being performed correctly. If it was performed correctly omit this exercise from your conditioning program.

- When performing the strength training exercises start by executing one to two sets of each exercise you select.
- After exercising a week, sets can be increased up to two to four.
- With most strength training exercises, perform between eight to fifteen repetitions in a set.
- If an exercise can not be performed with proper form for eight repetitions chances are the weight used is too heavy.
- If an exercise can be performed with proper form for more than fifteen repetitions the weight is probably too light.

This rule of thumb should give you an idea of how much weight should be used with each exercise.

The exercises that do not incorporate external resistance (dumbbells and barbells) such as abdominal exercises, push-ups, pull-ups and low back exercises can increase in intensity by increasing the repetitions. These exercises may have sets of ten to thirty repetitions in each set. In the case of push-ups, if a person is able to perform thirty repetitions on the knees this would indicate that he or she is ready to perform the exercise on the toes. If a person can perform thirty repetitions of push-ups on the toes then the are ready for plyometric push-ups.

It is a good idea to change the list of exercises on a regular basis so the muscles do not get too accustomed to the same movement. The more variety in a strength workout the more different types of demand are placed upon the muscles, forcing them to strengthen in a number of ways. **Try changing the list of exercises each week or every other week.** It is okay to repeat some of the same exercises but be sure to alternate at least two or three exercises.

The same approach should be taken in regards to endurance training. By alternating between different cardiovascular exercises the body is being challenged to meet many different types of movement. This can help reduce the chance of experiencing a plateau in the training program. A plateau is when the body does not seem to be developing at the same rate it had recently been.

When designing the endurance portion of the program remember to also start slowly and progress to higher intensity in a methodical manner. Start with ten to twenty minutes two to three times a week and slowly add five to ten minutes each week or add an additional day.

In regards to the flexibility portion of the program this should be performed daily even if the other parts of the program are not being performed on that day.

Flexibility is the key ingredient to prevent injuries. The strength training and endurance programs have a tendency to tighten the muscles so it is therefore essential that a person spend a considerable amount of time stretching the body back out. Although it is important to have a proper warm-up when exercising, most gains in flexibility will be received when stretches are performed after the strength and endurance workouts. **So be sure to take time at the end of each workout to properly cool down via stretching.**

One more note on strength training: in the next few pages, examples of a surfer's strength training & conditioning program will be given. There will also be examples of a home based program. The weights should be replaced with the proper amount according to your personal strength levels. It is important to understand that when performing the strength workout the exercises incorporate all of the major muscle groups of the body. If you intend to perform strength workouts more than three to four times a week it may be better to focus on the upper body on one day and the lower body on a different day.

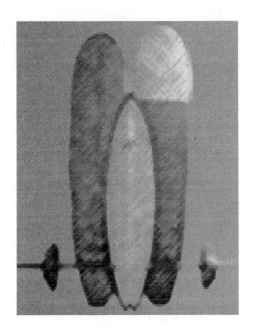

CHAPTER 8: WORKOUT LOG

Below is a list of all the strength, endurance, and flexibility exercises mentioned in this book. They are sectioned into different categories to make it easier to refer to when designing your own conditioning program.

Strength Exercises

Upper Body (Choose 3 to 5 exercises below)
- Push Up on Knees
- Push Up on Toes
- Push Up on Balance Board
- Plyometric Push Up on Balance Board
- Popping Push Up
- Burpees
- Bench Press
- Bench Dip
- Lat Pulldown
- Pull Up
- Horizontal Pull Up
- Straight Arm Pulldown
- Dumbbell Pullover
- One Arm Row
- Reverse Dumbbell Fly
- Triceps Pushdown
- External Rotation

Lower Body (Choose 3 to 5 exercises below)
- Bodyweight Squat
- Barbell Squat
- Dumbbell Squat
- Bodyweight Split Squat
- Barbell Split Squat
- Dumbbell Split Squat
- Bodyweight Forward Lunge
- Barbell Forward Lunge

- Dumbbell Forward Lunge
- Bodyweight Reverse Lunge
- Barbell Reverse Lunge
- Dumbbell Reverse Lunge
- Bodyweight Walking Lunge
- Barbell Walking Lunge
- Dumbbell Walking Lunge
- Wall Sit

Trunk & Torso (Choose 2 to 4 exercises below)
- Abdominal Crunch
- Oblique Crunch
- Low Back Exercise
- Hanging Leg Lift
- Supine Eagles

Endurance Exercises

- Longboard Paddling
- Shortboard Paddling
- Longboard Paddling with Resistance Bucket
- Shortboard Paddling with Resistance Bucket
- Partner Towing on Longboard
- Partner Towing on Shortboard
- Land Paddle with Resistance Band
- Walking
- Running
- Stair Climbing
- Rowing Machine

Flexibility Exercises

- Crossed Knee Lift
- Crossover Twist
- Mad Cat Stretch
- Chest & Shoulder Stretch

- Crossed Arm Stretch
- Arm Circles
- Shoulder Pivots
- Lateral Neck Stretch
- Forward Neck Stretch
- Downward Facing Dog
- Quadriceps Stretch

Home Workout

Week: #1 & #2	Set 1	Set 2	Set 3
Exercises	Wt./ Rep.	Wt./ Rep.	Wt./ Rep.
Ab Crunch	20reps	20reps	25 reps
Oblique Crunch	20reps	20reps	25 reps
Push-Ups (knees)	15 reps	15 reps	15 reps
Burpees	15 reps	15 reps	15 reps
Horiz. Pull Up	15 reps	12 reps	10 reps
Reverse Fly	5/15	5/15	5/15
Bodywt. Squat	15 reps	15 reps	15 reps
Forward Lunge	10 reps	10 reps	10 reps
Endurance	Dur.	Int.	Freq.
Paddle (longbd.)	20 min.	Med.	2x/wk.
Walking	30 min.	Low	2x/wk.

Flexibility (Perform Daily)			
Cr. Knee Lift	30 sec.		
Crossover Twist	30 sec.		
Mad Cat Str.	30 sec.		
Lat. Neck Str.	30 sec.		
For. Neck Str.	30 sec.		

Home Workout

Week: #3 & #4	Set 1	Set 2	Set 3
Exercises	Wt./ Rep.	Wt./ Rep.	Wt./ Rep.
Oblique Crunch	25 reps	25 reps	25 reps
Low Back Ex.	20 reps	20 reps	20 reps
Push-Ups (toes)	15 reps	15 reps	15 reps
Bench Dip	15 reps	15 reps	15 reps
D.B. Pullover	10/15	12/15	15/15
Ext. Rotation	5/15	5/15	5/15
Bwt. Split Squat	15 reps	15 reps	15 reps
Reverse Lunge	15 reps	15 reps	15 reps
Wall Sit	30 sec.	30 sec.	30 sec.
Endurance	Dur.	Int.	Freq.
Paddle (shortbd.)	20 min.	Med.	3x/wk.
Stairs	20 min.	Med.	2x/wk.

Flexibility (Perform Daily)			
Cr. Knee Lift	30 sec.		
Crossover Twist	30 sec.		
Mad Cat Str.	30 sec.		
Lat. Neck Str.	30 sec.		
For. Neck Str.	30 sec.		

Home Workout

Week: #5 & #6	Set 1	Set 2	Set 3
Exercises	Wt./ Rep.	Wt./ Rep.	Wt./ Rep.
Ab Crunch	25reps	25reps	25 reps
Supine Eagles	20reps	20reps	20 reps
Pop. Push-Ups	15 reps	15 reps	15 reps
Burpees	10 reps	12 reps	15 reps
Horiz. Pull Up	15 reps	15 reps	15 reps
Reverse Fly	5/15	5/15	8/15
Dumbbell Squat	10/15	15/12	20/10
Wall Sit	45 sec.	45 sec.	45 sec.
Endurance	Dur.	Int.	Freq.
Paddle w/ Pail (lgbd.)	30 min.	High	3x/wk.
Running	30 min.	Med.	2x/wk.

Flexibility (Perform Daily)			
Cr. Knee Lift	30 sec.		
Crossover Twist	30 sec.		
Mad Cat Str.	30 sec.		
Arm Circles	45 sec.		
Shoulder Pivots	45 sec.		

Home Workout

Week: #7 & #8	Set 1	Set 2	Set 3
Exercises	Wt./ Rep.	Wt./ Rep.	Wt./ Rep.
Low Back	20 reps	20 reps	20 reps
Ab Crunch	30 reps	30 reps	30 reps
Hanging Leg Lift	20 reps	20 reps	20 reps
Push Up/Bal. Bd.	10 reps	10 reps	10 reps
Bench Dips	20 reps	15 reps	10 reps
Pull Ups	10 reps	8 reps	8 reps
D.B. Pullover	10/15	15/12	20/10
Bwt. Split Squat	15 reps	15 reps	15 reps
Reverse Lunge	15 reps	15 reps	15 reps
Dumbbell Squat	15/15	20/12	20/12
Endurance	Dur.	Int.	Freq.
Partner Paddle	10/1 min.	High	2x/wk.
Stairs	25 min.	Med.	2x/wk.
Underwater Swim	10/20 sec.	Med.	2x/wk.

Flexibility (Perform Daily)			
Cr. Knee Lift	30 sec.	Dward. Dog	45 sec.
Crossover Twist	30 sec.		
Mad Cat Str.	30 sec.		
Cross. Arm Str.	45 sec.		
Shoulder Pivots	45 sec.		

Home Workout

Week: #9 & #10	Set 1	Set 2	Set 3
Exercises	Wt./ Rep.	Wt./ Rep.	Wt./ Rep.
Hanging Leg Lift	20 reps	25 reps	25 reps
Supine Eagles	30 reps	30 reps	30 reps
Ab Crunch	30 reps	30 reps	30 reps
Plyo. Push Up	10 reps	10 reps	10 reps
Burpees	20 reps	15 reps	10 reps
Reverse Fly	10/15	10/15	10/15
External Rotation	5/15	5/15	5/15
Wall Sit	1 min.	1 min.	1 min.
Walking Lunge	20 reps	20 reps	20 reps
Endurance	Dur.	Int.	Freq.
Paddle w/ Pail (shbd.)	10/ 1min.	High	2x/wk.
Running	40 min.	Med.	2x/wk.
Underwater Swim	10/ 30sec.	Med.	2x/wk.

Flexibility   (Perform Daily)

Arm Circles	1 min.	Lat. Neck Str.	45 sec.
Shoulder Pivots	1 min.	Dward. Dog	1 min.
Quad Stretch	45 sec.		
Mad Cat Str.	1 min.		
For. Neck Str.	45 sec.		

Gym Workout

Week: #1 & #2	Set 1	Set 2	Set 3
Exercises	Wt./ Rep.	Wt./ Rep.	Wt./ Rep.
Ab Crunch	20 reps	20 reps	20 reps
Oblique Crunch	20 reps	20 reps	20 reps
Push Up (knees)	15 reps	15 reps	15 reps
D.B. Bench Press	15/15	20/12	20/10
Lat Pulldown	60/15	70/12	80/10
External Rotation	5/15	5/15	5/15
Dumbbell Squat	15/15	20/12	20/10
Bwt. Split Squat	15 reps	15 reps	15 reps
Endurance	Dur.	Int.	Freq.
Paddle Lgbd.	20 min.	Med.	2x/wk.
Walking	30 min.	Low	2x/wk.

Flexibility (Perform Daily)

Cr. Knee Lift	30 sec.		
Crossover Twist	30 sec.		
Mad Cat Str.	30 sec.		
For. Neck Str.	30 sec.		
Lat. Neck Str.	30 sec.		

Gym Workout

Week: #3 & #4	Set 1	Set 2	Set 3
Exercises	Wt./ Rep.	Wt./ Rep.	Wt./ Rep.
Ab Crunch	20 reps	25 reps	30 reps
Supine Eagles	20 reps	20 reps	20 reps
Push Up (toes)	15 reps	15 reps	15 reps
Bench Press (bar)	50/15	60/12	70/10
Str. Arm Pdown.	20/15	25/12	30/10
D.B. Pullover	10/15	15/15	20/12
External Rotation	5/15	5/15	5/15
Squat (barbell)	60/15	70/12	80/10
Split Squat (bar)	20/15	30/12	40/10
Endurance	Dur.	Int.	Freq.
Paddle (longboard)	30 min.	Med.	2x/wk.
Running	30 min.	Med.	2x/wk.

Flexibility   (Perform Daily)

Arm Circles	30 sec.	
Shoulder Pivots	30 sec.	
Cross. Knee Lift	30 sec.	
Crossover Twist	30 sec.	
Mad Cat Str.	30 sec.	

Gym Workout

Week: #5 & #6	Set 1	Set 2	Set 3
Exercises	Wt./ Rep.	Wt./ Rep.	Wt./ Rep.
Oblique Crunch	25 reps	25 reps	25 reps
Low Back Ex.	20 reps	20 reps	20 reps
Push Up (Bal. Bd.)	15 reps	15 reps	15 reps
Bench Dips	15 reps	15 reps	15 reps
Horiz. Pull Up	15 reps	12 reps	10 reps
One Arm Row	15/15	20/12	25/10
Walking Lunge	20 reps	20 reps	20 reps
Dumbbell Squat	15/15	20/15	25/12
Wall Sit	1 min.	30 sec.	30 sec.
Endurance	Dur.	Int.	Freq.
Paddle (shortboard)	30 min.	Med.	2x/wk.
Stairs	20 min.	Med.	2x/wk.
Flexibility (Perform Daily)			
Cr. Arm Stretch	30 sec.		
Chest/Shoulder	30 sec.		
Cr. Knee Lift	45 sec.		
Crossover Twist	45 sec.		
Mad Cat Str.	45 sec.		

Gym Workout

Week: #7 & #8	Set 1	Set 2	Set 3
Exercises	Wt./ Rep.	Wt./ Rep.	Wt./ Rep.
Hanging Leg Lift	20 reps	25 reps	25 reps
Ab Crunch	30 reps	30 reps	30 reps
Pop. Push Up	12 reps	12 reps	12 reps
Burpees	12 reps	12 reps	12 reps
Pull Up	12 reps	12 reps	10 reps
Reverse Fly	8/15	10/12	15/10
D.B. Walk. Lunge	10/16	15/12	20/10
Rev. Lunge (bar)	bar/15	10/12	20/10
Split Squat (bar)	bar/15	10/12	20/8
Endurance	Dur.	Int.	Freq.
Paddle w/ Pail	20 min.	High	2x/wk.
Rowing	20 min.	Med.	2x/wk.
Underwater Swim	10/ 30sec.	Med.	2x/wk.

Flexibility   (Perform Daily)

Cr. Knee Lift	1 min.	
Crossover Twist	1 min.	
Mad Cat Str.	45 sec.	
Dward. Dog	1 min.	
Lat. Neck Str.	45 sec.	

Gym Workout

Week: #9 & #10	Set 1	Set 2	Set 3
Exercises	Wt./ Rep.	Wt./ Rep.	Wt./ Rep.
Hanging Leg Lift	30 reps	30 reps	30 reps
Supine Eagles	30 reps	30 reps	30 reps
Ab Crunch	30 reps	30 reps	30 reps
Plyo. Push Up	12 reps	12 reps	12 reps
Bench Press (bar)	80/15	90/12	100/10
Lat Pulldown	60/15	70/15	80/15
Tricep Pushdown	20/15	25/15	30/12
Wall Sit	1 min.	1 min.	1 min.
Split Squat (d.b.)	10/16	15/12	20/10
Squat (Barbell)	60/15	75/12	90/10
Endurance	Dur.	Int.	Freq.
Partner Paddle	10/ 1min.	High	2x/wk.
Swim	40 min.	Med.	2x/wk.
Underwater Swim	10/ 30sec.	Med.	2x/wk.

Flexibility (Perform Daily)			
Arm Circles	1 min.	Lat. Neck Str.	45 sec.
Shoulder Pivots	1 min.	Dward. Dog	1 min.
Quad Stretch	45 sec.		
Mad Cat Str.	1 min.		
For. Neck Str.	45 sec.		

Fit To Surf

My Workout

Week:	Set 1	Set 2	Set 3
Exercises	Wt./ Rep.	Wt./ Rep.	Wt./ Rep.
Endurance	Dur.	Int.	Freq.

Flexibility   (Perform Daily)

My Workout

Week:	Set 1	Set 2	Set 3
Exercises	Wt./ Rep.	Wt./ Rep.	Wt./ Rep.

Endurance	Dur.	Int.	Freq.

Flexibility   (Perform Daily)

My Workout

Week:	Set 1	Set 2	Set 3
Exercises	Wt./ Rep.	Wt./ Rep.	Wt./ Rep.
Endurance	Dur.	Int.	Freq.

Flexibility (Perform Daily)

My Workout

Week:	Set 1	Set 2	Set 3
Exercises	Wt./ Rep.	Wt./ Rep.	Wt./ Rep.
Endurance	Dur.	Int.	Freq.

Flexibility (Perform Daily)

My Workout

Week:	Set 1	Set 2	Set 3
Exercises	Wt./ Rep.	Wt./ Rep.	Wt./ Rep.
Endurance	Dur.	Int.	Freq.

Flexibility   (Perform Daily)

My Workout

Week:	Set 1	Set 2	Set 3
Exercises	Wt./ Rep.	Wt./ Rep.	Wt./ Rep.

Endurance	Dur.	Int.	Freq.

Flexibility   (Perform Daily)

Fit To Surf

My Workout

Week:	Set 1	Set 2	Set 3
Exercises	Wt./ Rep.	Wt./ Rep.	Wt./ Rep.
Endurance	Dur.	Int.	Freq.

Flexibility (Perform Daily)

My Workout

Week:	Set 1	Set 2	Set 3
Exercises	Wt./ Rep.	Wt./ Rep.	Wt./ Rep.

Endurance	Dur.	Int.	Freq.

Flexibility (Perform Daily)

My Workout

Week:	Set 1	Set 2	Set 3
Exercises	Wt./ Rep.	Wt./ Rep.	Wt./ Rep.
Endurance	Dur.	Int.	Freq.

Flexibility   (Perform Daily)

My Workout

Week:	Set 1	Set 2	Set 3
Exercises	Wt./ Rep.	Wt./ Rep.	Wt./ Rep.

Endurance	Dur.	Int.	Freq.

Flexibility   (Perform Daily)

My Workout

Week:	Set 1	Set 2	Set 3
Exercises	Wt./ Rep.	Wt./ Rep.	Wt./ Rep.
Endurance	Dur.	Int.	Freq.

Flexibility   (Perform Daily)

For More Information
on
Strength Training & Conditioning:

Body Balance and Postural Realignment
Web Site: www.dpdc-mbf.com
or Dynamics Of Physical Development Consultants
1840 41st Avenue #102-141
Capitola, CA. 95010
(831) 685-8211

The 7-Minute Rotator Cuff Solution. by Joseph Horrigan, D.C. and Jerry Robinson

Sport Stretch. by Michael J. Alter

Essentials of Strength Training & Conditioning. by Thomas R. Baechle and Roger W. Earle

Quick Order Form

Please send check or money order to:
Emerson Publishing Co.
551 37ᵗʰ Ave. Santa Cruz, Ca. 95062

Fit To Surf:
A Surfer's Guide To Strength Training & Conditioning
$18.95 (includes shipping & handling)

Please allow 4-6 weeks for delivery.

Name: _____

Street Address: _____ Apt. _____

City: _____ State: ____ Zip: _____

Email Address: _____